Ahmed HARBAOUI

Management of acute tumor-induced hydrocephalus

Ahmed HARBAOUI

Management of acute tumor-induced hydrocephalus

The nurse's role

ScienciaScripts

Cover image: www.ingimage.com

This book is a translation from the original published under ISBN 978-620-6-72550-3.

Publisher:
Sciencia Scripts
is a trademark of
Dodo Books Indian Ocean Ltd. and OmniScriptum S.R.L publishing group

120 High Road, East Finchley, London, N2 9ED, United Kingdom
Str. Armeneasca 28/1, office 1, Chisinau MD-2012, Republic of Moldova, Europe
Printed at: see last page
ISBN: 978-620-8-20613-0

TABLE OF CONTENTS

INTRODUCTION

Hydrocephalus is defined as an abnormal accumulation of CSF in the fluid cavities of the brain under a regime of high pressure at a given time in its evolution. It is a frequent pathology in neurological and neurosurgical settings [1].

It is caused by dilation of the ventricular system. It is often secondary to an obstruction in the CSF circulation pathways (obstructive hydrocephalus) but may also be secondary to CSF secretion or resorption disorders (communicating hydrocephalus) [1].

In Tunisia, the incidence of hydrocephalus is estimated at 5.24% of the population.all central nervous system malformations [1].It is a condition with multiple aetiologies which differ according to age and which are dominated by malformations, infections and tumours. [1]

Hydrocephalus is a neurosurgical emergency, which can be life-threatening due to the intracranial hypertension it causes. It is even more serious when it is secondary to a brain tumour. The aim of this study was to find out about the different therapeutic methods for acute hydrocephalus of tumour origin and the role of nurses in its management.

MATERIALS AND METHODS

I. Equipment

1. Place of the survey

This survey was carried out in the neurosurgery department of the main military training hospital in Tunis.

2. Survey period

The data collection period was 1 month.

3. Patients

This is a retrospective study based on the withdrawal of 32 records of patients having been treated for tumour hydrocephalus, collected over a period of 10 and a half years from 2009 to 2019.

- Inclusion criteria

Our study includes any patient with acute hydrocephalus of tumour confirmed by neuroimaging.

- Exclusion criteria

Our study excludes any patient presenting with acute hydrocephalus that is not of tumour origin, brain tumour is not associated with hydrocephalus and files that lack the necessary data to make the study.

II. Methodology

1. Data collection

To collect the data, we drew up a data collection medium (see Appendix 1), which is a form containing the variables measured to achieve the objectives set. We selected the following variables:

- Age
- Sex
- Time to diagnosis
- Clinical signs
- Type of neuroimaging
- Type of intervention

2. Processing data

- The data collected is processed on a microcomputer.
- Thecharts and tables are onEXCEL under WINDOWS.

RESULTS

I. Epidemiological data

1) Breakdown by gender

There is a slight male predominance, with a sex ratio of 1.5 (Figure 1).

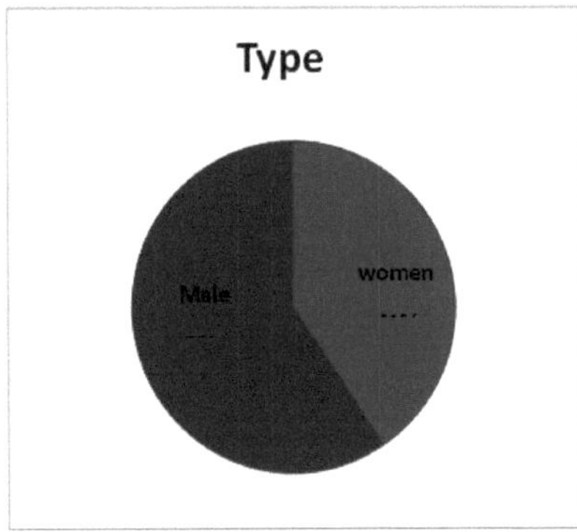

Figure 1: Breakdown by gender

2) Breakdown of patients by age at discovery

- We divided our patients into three age groups (Figure 2)
- According to the diagram, the majority of our patients were in the age group [0-6 years].

• The average age of our population was 14.

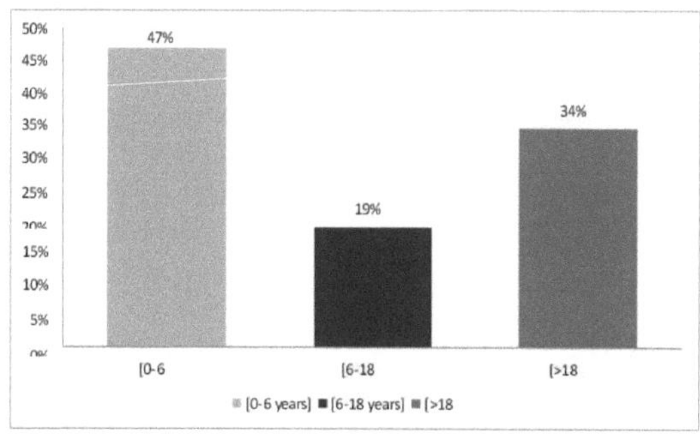

Figure 2: Breakdown by age of discovery

II.DATA CLINICAL

1) Delay diagnosis

Between a minimum of 02 days and a maximum of 60 days.

2) Clinical signs

Clinical signs are dominated by an HTIC syndrome (headache, vomiting and visual disturbance).

Table I: Breakdown by clinical signs

Consciousness disorder	7	12.5%
HTIC syndrome	30	93.75%
Convulsion	5	15.63%
Impairment of the VIème cranial pair	2	6.25%

III. PARA CLINICAL DATA

1) Type of neuro- imaging

- Cerebral CT scans were performed in 29 patients.

- Brain MRI was performed in 18 patients, including 3 who underwent MRI at the outset (Figure 3)

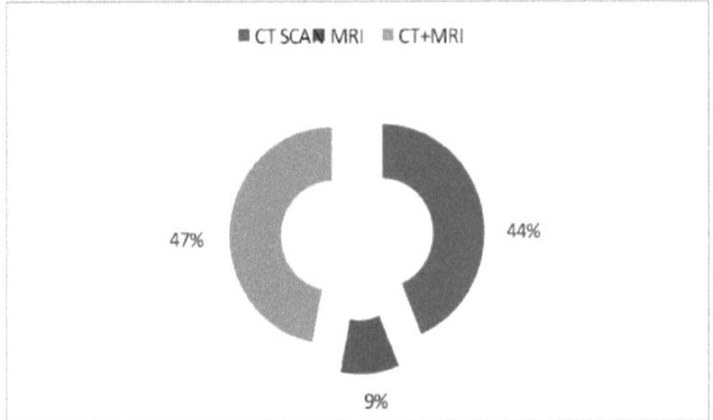

Figure 3: breakdown by neuroimaging

2) Tumour site

- The tumour site most affected was sub-tentorial. (Figure 4).

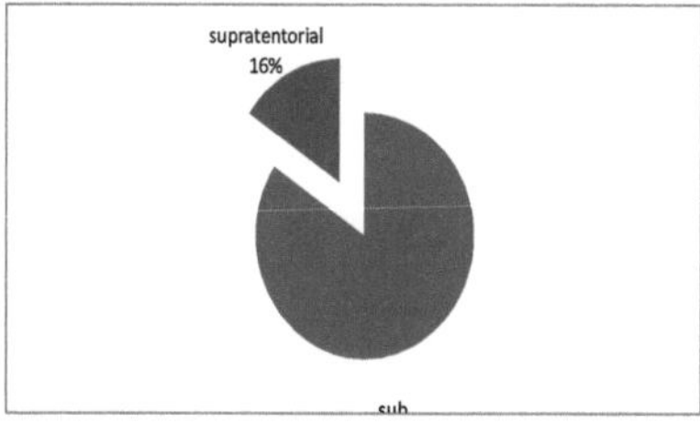

Figure 4: Distribution by tumour site

- The majority of these tumours were in V4 (Figure 5).

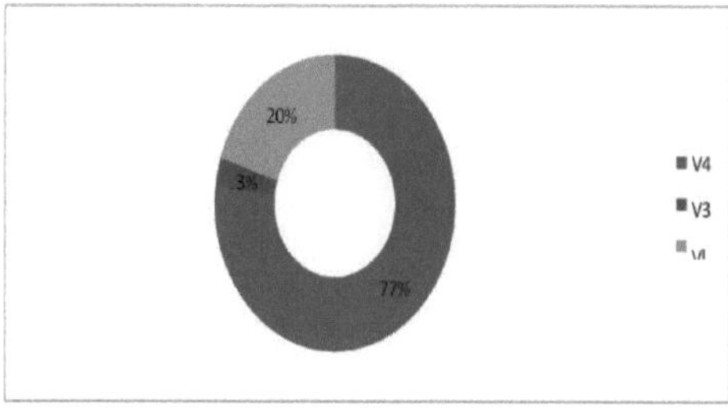

Figure 5: Distribution according to tumour location

The type of hydrocephalus

- tri-ventricular hydrocephalus is predominant (Figure 6)

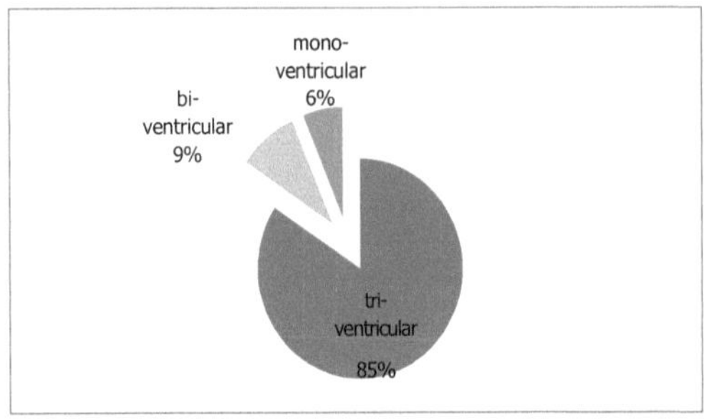

Figure 6: Distribution according to type of hydrocephalus

IV. Treatment

All cases were treated surgically, with tumour removal in each case.

• 13 patients underwent ventriculoperitoneal shunting (PVS), i.e.

41%

• 5 patients benefited from an external ventricular bypass (EVB), i.e.

16%

• 4 patients have had a ventriculocisternostomy (VCSE) by endoscopy

(13%)

• 10 patients underwent immediate tumour excision (30%)

Table 3: Breakdown by treatment

DVE	5
DVP	13
VCSE	4
Initial tumour removal	10

V. Evolution

The evolution of the hydrocephalus was favourable in 100% of cases, with clinical improvement (regression of signs of HTIC) and/or radiological improvement (reduction in ventricular dilatation on cerebral CT).

VI. Complications

In our work, we were able to find :

• 8 cases of bacterial meningitis

• 1 case of valve blockage

• 1 case of extra-ventricular displacement of the DVE ventricular catheter

• 1 case of failed VCSE requiring DVP

DISCUSSION

I. Epidemiological data

1. Type

Most studies of hydrocephalus of tumour origin show a male predominance, with a sex ratio generally greater than 1.5 [2].

In our study, we found 19 male patients (59%) and 13 female patients (41%), with a slight male predominance and a sex ratio of 1.5.

2. Age

In the literature, the average age of discovery of a brain tumour complicated by hydrocephalus is around 5 to 10 years in children [3,4] and around 36 years in adults [5]. In our series, the age group most affected was 0 to 6 years in 15 cases. cases (47%) with an average age of 14 years.

II. Data

1. Delay diagnosis

The time taken to diagnose the disease varies greatly from one series to another. It can range from a few days to a few weeks. It was even several months to 1 year for CHTIRA et al [6]. In our study, the time to diagnosis ranged from a minimum of 02 days to a maximum of 60 days.

2. Clinical signs

According to BERETTE et al, the frequency of HTIC in hydrocephalus associated with a posterior fossa tumour was 92.5% [7], which is consistent with our study (present in 93.75% of cases). In addition to the HTIC syndrome, hydrocephalus of tumour origin can produce :

- consciousness disorders (12.5% in our study).

- convulsions (15.63% in our study).

- involvement of the VIème cranial pair (6.25% in our study).

- Behavioural and character disorders

- cerebellar syndrome, ataxia on walking, nystagmus, dysarthria and/or coordination disorders, and signs of pyramidal irritation. [8]

III. PARA-CLINICAL DATA

1. Type of neuroimaging

A cerebral CT scan shows the entire ventricular system and gives an idea of the aetiology of the hydrocephalus. By showing the characteristics of ventricular dilatation (uni-, bi- or tri-ventricular) in the event of an obstruction, the CT scan makes it possible to locate the site of the obstacle.In our series, the first additional examination to be carried out in the presence of intracranial hypertension is a cerebral CT scan. This was performed in 29 patients.**Cerebral MRI** offers better image resolution than CT scans, avoids the need to irradiate patients and is more sensitive for exploring small tumours of the central nervous system or cerebral malformations that may be the cause of hydrocephalus. MRI Cerebral CT, rarely used as a first-line examination (in 3 cases in our series), is often used as a complement to cerebral CT (18 cases in our series).

2. Tumour site

Tumours of the posterior cerebral fossa are responsible for obstructive hydrocephalus in more than 80% of cases [9,10]. This was also the case in our study, where the tumour site most affected was subtentorial (posterior cerebral fossa) in (84%) compared with the supratentorial site (16%). The majority of these tumours were intraventricular (V4 in 23 patients, VL in 6 patients and V3 in 1 patient).

IV. Treatment

Therapeutic management of acute hydrocephalus of tumour origin must reduce intracranial pressure and restore free flow of CSF. Symptomatic medical treatment must therefore be started very quickly while awaiting surgical treatment, which will be symptomatic and then aetiological, or even aetiological from the outset.

1) Mannitol medical treatment

- It decreases cerebral water content by increasing osmolarity and reduces plasma viscosity, leading to compensatory cerebral vasoconstriction if the autoregulatory mechanisms are still preserved.

- Mannitol is also thought to reduce CSF secretion and volume.

- Mannitol is generally prescribed at a dose of 0.5 to 2 g/kg intravenously for 15 minutes, followed by boluses of 25 g as soon as the intracranial pressure rises.

- Possible side effects (renal failure, dehydration, rebound effect, etc.) should be taken into account [11].

Hyperventilation to reduce PCO2: in certain cases, the PaCO2 concentration can be lowered to 30-35 mmHg (increase in ventilator frequency). By inducing vasoconstriction, the aim is to reduce cerebral blood flow, and consequently cerebral blood volume and ICP [11].

30° pro-Trendelenburg position, head in line with the body It improves ICH[11].

Corticosteroids: These act on peritumoral oedema by reducing vascular permeability, which they reduce by their anti-inflammatory action, and reduce HTIC [11].

Furosemide: This diuretic could be combined with traditional corticosteroids in the hope of improving the anti-oedematous action. It is thought to increase and prolong the effect of mannitol [11].

2) Surgical treatment

2.1 Symptomatic surgical treatment :

This is the treatment for acute hydrocephalus proper. It consists of either external (temporary) or internal (permanent) ventricular drainage by ventriculoperitoneal shunt or endoscopic ventriculocisternostomy.

2.1.1 External ventricular bypass :

a) Description

The external ventricular shunt (EVS) consists of a multifenestrated catheter surgically implanted in one of the lateral ventricles, connected to an external tube containing a sterile graduated collection system **(Figure 7)**, which allows controlled, transient external drainage of CSF. By adjusting the height of the drainage device, you can control the flow of CSF. Drainage works on the principle of communicating vessels. It can be set up very quickly and is therefore best suited to extreme emergencies [12]. In our series, 5 patients benefited from this procedure (16%).

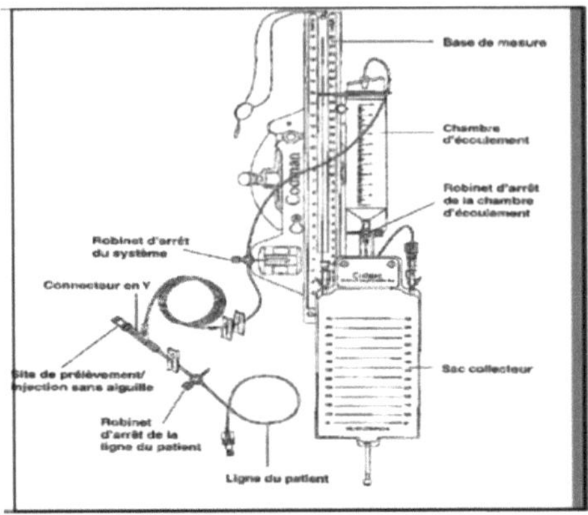

Figure7: illustration of the drainage system. [13]

b) Installing the drainage level

Level zero is defined by the ear's external auditory canal (EAC) and corresponds to Monroe's hole in the ventricular system. Back pressure is prescribed by doctors to control the flow of CSF. This counter-pressure is obtained by positioning the dropper chamber at the prescribed height (in cm H2O) in relation to the zero previously established.The CSF flows as a result of the pressure difference between the ventricles. and the drip chamber. It is therefore essential to comply with the prescribed level regardless of the patient's position (30°, half-seated, etc.), otherwise there is a risk that the drainage will be either too great or ineffective. [14] The 0 of the drainage system and the level of the pressure head must therefore always be at the same level (that of the ACE) and must be readjusted according to the position of the patient's head. (Figure 8)

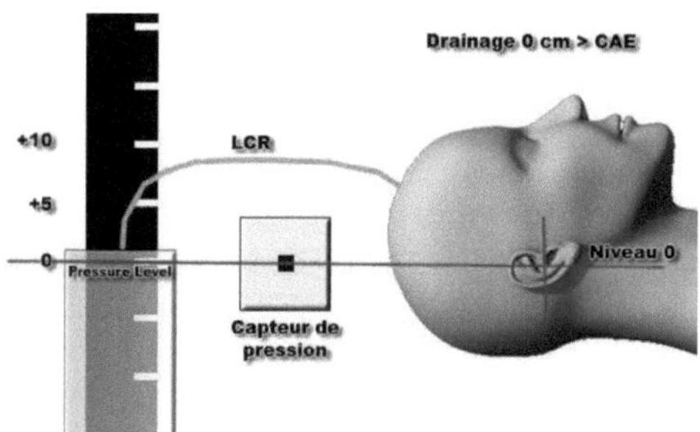

Figure 8: Theoretical representation of level 0

c) The risks

- Infectious ++++ (abscesses in the path of the drain, ventriculitis, meningitis, CSF leaks around the catheter): MANIPULATIONS MUST THEREFORE BE LIMITED AS MUCH AS POSSIBLE AND CARRIED OUT WITH EXTREMELY RIGOROUS ASEPSIS.

The drainage port and the beginning of the catheter must remain sterile and under an occlusive dressing.

- Haemorrhagic: intracerebral haematoma with or without ventricular flooding when the ventricular catheter is inserted.

- Malfunction :

- obstruction or migration of the ventricular catheter or too little drainage of the CSF, which can lead to HTIC

- over-drainage (hyper-drainage), which can lead to impaired alertness, intracerebral or especially subdural bleeding, or even cerebral involvement. [14]

2.1.2 Ventriculoperitoneal bypass

Ventriculoperitoneal (PVP) diversion of cerebrospinal fluid is the most commonly used treatment for hydrocephalus. [15]

a) Description

This technique consists of draining CSF from the ventricular cavities into the peritoneal cavity, where it is reabsorbed. This is done using a shunt system consisting of a ventricular catheter, a valve and a peritoneal catheter **(Figure 9)**[16]. In our series, 13 patients underwent ventriculo-peritoneal shunting (41%).

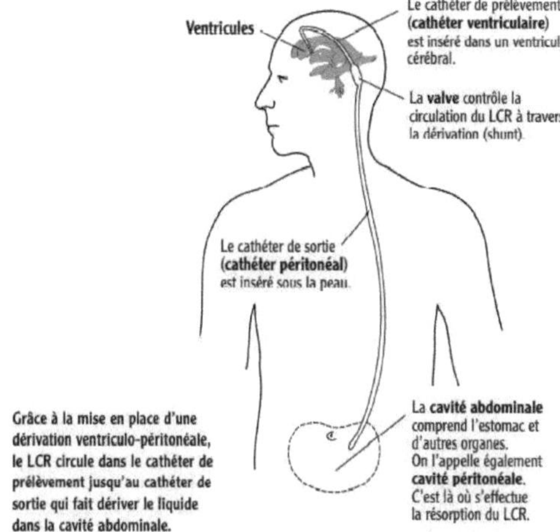

Figure 9: Components of a ventriculoperitoneal shunt

b) The risks

- obstruction (blockage of the bypass system)

- infection (meningitis)

- mechanical failure (rupture or dislocation of the bypass)

- excessive or ineffective drainage of CSF

- Gastrointestinal perforation[17].

2.1.3 Endoscopic ventirculo-cisternostomy

a) Description

Endoscopic ventriculocisternostomy (VCSE) involves establishing communication between the third ventricle and the basal cisterns using a ventriculoscope introduced through a drill hole. frontal. The stoma in the floor of the third ventricle is used to bypass an obstacle in the mesencephalic aqueduct. This is an internal bypass of the CSF. [18]**(Figure 10)**In our series, this technique was performed on 4 patients.

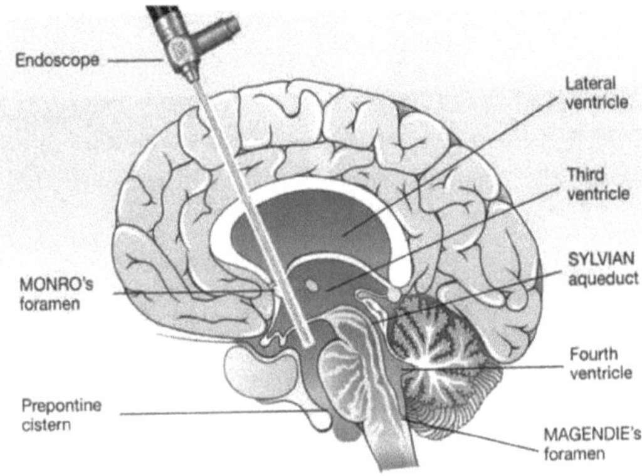

Figure 10: Theoretical representation of the VCS [19].

b) The risks

- Intraventricular haemorrhage

- Neurological disorders:Coma, disorders of the vigilance, convulsions, oculomotor impairment, memory disorders.

- Meningitis

2.2 Etiological surgical treatment

This is the radical treatment of the brain tumour itself. The tumour is removed as completely as possible, removing the excess tumour volume within the cranial cavity, which interferes with the free flow of CSF.In certain cases where acute hydrocephalus is not clearly life-threatening, and where surgical resection is possible within a short period of time, the patient may benefit from immediate tumour resection, which will ensure that the aetiological treatment and restoration of normal CSF circulation can be achieved within the same operating time. In our series, 10 patients (30%) underwent immediate tumour resection.

V. Complications

1. Meningitis :

Can complicate all types of valve. They may be classic purulent meningitis, but 60% are due to white staphylococcus, of cutaneous origin, with contamination occurring when the equipment is inserted, even when this is revealed late. These forms of meningitis develop quietly, manifesting as malfunctioning of the shunt system, persistent febrile symptoms or a slight deterioration in general condition. Diagnosis is based on lumbar puncture, which proves meningitis, but only with difficulty finds the germ, which is not very pathogenic. Treatment is difficult and relies on antibiotic therapy and 104 removal of the material; a temporary external bypass is sometimes necessary. The best treatment is preventive: the surgeon's experience, the speed of the operation, and the reduction in the size and number of skin incisions, Antibiotic therapy targeting white staphylococcus and the use of an operating theatre isolator. These measures have reduced the number of infectious complications to less than 5%[20]. In our study, 8 patients developed meningitis.

2. Valve obstruction

The second most likely site of obstruction is the shunt valve. The most common causes of valve obstruction include hardware failure and obstruction by tissue debris or blood products. There is currently no valve on the market that is less likely to obstruct than others[21] Regardless of which valve is inserted, there are a few simple steps that neurosurgeons can take to reduce the risk of valve obstruction preoperatively: Once the ventricular catheter is in place, it is suggested that a small amount of CSF be drained to remove blood and tissue debris before the valve is connected to the shunt system. In addition, when connecting the valve, it is recommended that the system be irrigated with saline, to prevent accidental introduction of blood or tissue debris into the catheters and valve. [22] In our study, only one patient presented with valve obstruction.

3. Migration

It is defined as the phenomenon whereby the catheter moves from its appropriate initial location to a position where drainage is severely compromised or absent. Ventricular catheter migration is It is often secondary to the existence of a mechanical force, particularly in young children who move their heads too abruptly. It can also be secondary to low resistance at the connection with the valve or, more rarely, to poor placement of the connection between the ventricular catheter and the valve[23]. In our study, only one patient had an extra-ventricular displacement of the ventricular catheter of the DVE.

VI. Nursing care

1. Pre-operative nursing care

Psychological preparation :

- Patients must be able to express their fears and lack of knowledge at any time.
- Establishing a relationship of trust will allow patients to express their anxieties and ask any questions they may have.

Skin preparation :

Aim: to reduce the risk of infection by reducing transient bacterial flora and commensal flora in the surgical area.

- Depilation : Shaving
- Shower: With antiseptic soap General preparation :

- Check the integrity of the file contents

- Light meal the evening before

- Fasting after midnight

- Taking vital parameters

- No preoperative anticoagulant The morning of the operation :

- Verification of biological and radiological examinations

- Fasting: remind the patient

- Final check of the file

- Reassuring them when they leave

2. Post-operative nursing care

a) DVE

General precautions

- Respect the prescribed level and maintain it whatever the patient's position.

- No injections or suction directly into the drain (unless prescribed by a doctor and must be carried out by a doctor)

- Close the clamps when moving the patient and reopen them as soon as possible.

Each time the system is mobilised, its level will change. If the DVE is not clamped, there are two risks:

- If the DVE is too low :

Risk of abrupt emptying of the CSF, leading to ventricular collapse

- If the DVE is too high :

Risk of HTIC and ventricular dilatation.

Nursing supervision

- Carry out neurological monitoring: A change in pupils, a change in the state of consciousness or the appearance of a neurological deficit should alert the nurse, who should seek medical advice.

- Monitor the appearance of the CSF: watery, haemorrhagic, cloudy, purulent ...

- Check that the system is watertight and permeable by lowering the dropper chamber below the ACE twice every 12 hours (for a few seconds).

- A check that the system is not folded or occluded is essential.

- Monitor the amount of CSF in the drip chamber every hour, every two hours or every four hours (depending on the prescription) and empty it into the collection bag each time. If the drainage flow rate changes abnormally (flow rate > 10-20cc/h or < 5cc/h), inform the doctor.

- record the amount of CSF on the monitoring sheet provided.

- Temperature should be monitored on a twice-daily basis: any hyperthermia should raise the suspicion of meningitis.

- Changing the dressing will allow regular monitoring of the puncture site, the catheter and the surgical wound. This should be done every 48 hours, using rigorous asepsis.

- Monitoring of decubitus-related complications. [13]

b) DVP, VCSE and immediate tumour removal

Neurological monitoring :

- State of consciousness

- Signs of HTIC: headache, vomiting and visual disturbance

- Look for sensory or motor disorders to detect a compressive haematoma or CSF leak.

- Testing sensitivity

- Testing motor skills

- Sphincter control Haemodynamic monitoring :

- Pulse

- Blood pressure

- Temperature: strict, regular monitoring to detect the risk of infection

- Respiratory rate Diuresis monitoring

Pain monitoring: in order to adapt the analgesic treatment and make it more effective. modified by the doctor if necessary

Dressing change: to prevent infection or clot formation, protect the wound, help healing and ensure patient comfort and hygiene.

- As prescribed by your doctor (generally every 48 hours)

- Observe rigorous asepsis

- Monitor the puncture site every time it is dressed and report any pain, redness, swelling or warmth to detect the risk of infection.

- The dressing must be occlusive, sterile and clean at all times

Monitoring complications associated with decubitus :

- Changing positions to prevent pressure sores and monitoring the position of the head to avoid pressure on the valve.

- Ensure nutritional balance.

Biological monitoring: on medical prescription

Nursing care:

- Help with washing for certain patients.

- Bed refurbishment, bed hygiene.

- Helping some patients to eat their meals.

CONCLUSION

This study is part of a theoretical and practical study carried out at the main military training hospital in Tunis, and more specifically in the neurosurgery department. The subject of this work is hydrocephalus of tumoral origin.This hospital-based study looked at the different treatment methods for tumour-induced hydrocephalus and clarified the role of nurses in the management of this pathological condition. Acute hydrocephalus of tumour origin affects all age groups and more specifically children.The clinical signs of acute tumour hydrocephalus are dominated by the HTIC syndrome. The tumour sites most affected were subentorally and in the fourth ventricle. Tumour removal was performed in all cases. Nurses play a vital role in this pathology, and must master the specific gestures and attitudes required to participate effectively in progress in the neurosurgery department. They are also responsible for the psychological care and support of patients' families and relatives.

APPENDICES

Data collection form (appendix 1)

Epidemiological data :

- Gender :male female
- Age of discovery :

o Ages 0-6

o 6y-18y

o >18 years

Clinical data :

- Diagnosis time:
- Clinical signs :

o Consciousness disorder

o HTIC syndrome

o Convulsion

o Impairment of the VIème cranial pair

Para-clinical data :

Type of neuroimaging :

- CT SCAN
- MRI
- CT+MRI

- Tumour site :
  - sus tentoriel
  - Sub tentorial
- Tumour location :
  - V3
  - V4
  - VL
- Type of hydrocephalus :
  - Single ventricular
  - Bi-ventricular
  - Tri-ventricular

Treatment :

- Initial tumour removal
- DVE
- DVP
- VCSE

Trend: favourablefavourable

Complication

BIBLIOGRAPHICAL REFERENCES

1. Dominic NPT. Hydrocephalus. Neurosurgery 2009;27(3):130-4.

2. MICHEAL D. TAYLOR, JAMES T. RUTKA. Medulloblastoma.

3. LACOUR B, DESANDES E, MALLOL N, SOMMELET D.The Lorraine childhood cancer register: incidence, survival 1983-.1999.Archives de pediatrie 2005;12:1577-86.

4. ROGER J. PACKER. Brain tumors in children. Arch Neurol. 1999;56: 421-5

5. LEZAR S, ZAMIATI W, HASSAN H, ADIL A.Les tumeurs de la fosse cerebrale posterieure (a propos de 80 cas). EMC (Elsevier Masson SAS),Neurologie, 2008;89(10):1580-1.

6. DR.KAMEL CHTIRA, Treatment of hydrocephalus due to tumours of the posterior cerebral fossa: ventriculoperitoneal diversion versus ventriculocisternostomy.

7. BERETE I. Tumours of the posterior cerebral fossa. Thesis Medicine. Fez 2009

8. CAIRE F, GUEYE EM, FISCHER-LOKOU D, DURAND A, MARTEL BONCOEUR MP, FAURE PA, et al.

Hydrocephalus in children and adults. EMC (Elsevier Masson SAS), Neurology, 17-160-C-40, 2009.

9. CHERQAOUI A H.Neoplasms of the posterior cerebral fossa in adults.These de Med. Casablanca 1992,19.

10. KHASAWNEH NH.Hydrocephalus in posterior fossa tumours: Ventriculoperitoneal shunt versus endoscopic third ventriculostomy.Pan Arab Journal of Neurosurgery 2010; 14(1):46-9.

11. https://www.oncolie.fr/espace-medecins/les-referentiels/classement-anatomy/nervous system/neuro-oncology-treatment-symptoms/f

12. file:///C:/Users/LENOVO/Downloads/SARI%20DONMEZ_These med_2016.pdf

13. https://www.srlf.org/metier-dide-reanimation/fiches-techniques/fiche-n11-external-ventricular-derivation/

14. file:///C:/Users/LENOVO/Downloads/protocole_dve_2017%20(2).pdf

15. http://dvpdumonde.org/images/webneurologie.pdf

16. http://infoneuro.mcgill.ca/images/stories/Documents/vp_shunfr.pdf

17. Mr. Aristide MBONIHANKUYE. Complications of

ventriculoperitoneal shunts in hydrocephalus.

18. http://wd.fmpm.uca.ma/biblio/theses/annee-htm/FT/2009/these26-09.pdf

19. GUIOT G.Ventriculo-cisternostomy for stenosis of the aqueduct of Sylvius.Acta Neurochir (Wien) 1973;28:275-89.

20. P . Landrieu , J. Comoy, M. Zerah Hydrocephalus in children EMC 1988 Pediatrics - Infectious diseases [4-096-A-10]

21. Hiroji MIYAKE. Shunt Devices for the Treatment of Adult Hydrocephalus: Recent Progress and Characteristics. Neurologia medico-chirurgica Advance Publication Date: April 4, 2016

22. Browd SR, Ragel BT, Gottfried ON, Kestle JRW. Failure of Cerebrospinal Fluid Shunts: Part I: Obstruction and Mechanical Failure. PediatrNeurol 2006;34:83- 92.

23. Strachan R, Woon K, wong P, taylor J. Pitfalls in perinatal shunt surgery: A personal perspective. Eur J PediatrSurg 2002;12:S25-S52.

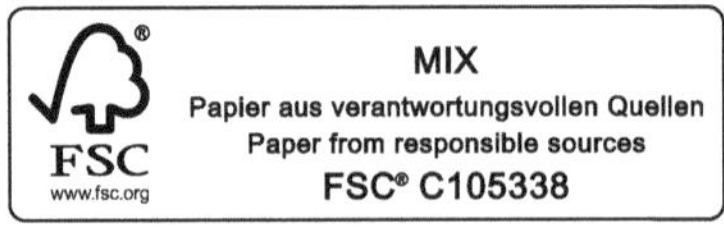

Printed by Books on Demand GmbH, Norderstedt / Germany